NAVIGATING TONGUE TIE WITH CONFIDENCE AND CARE

Unlocking The Secrets And Discovering Resilience For Empowering Parents With Expert Guidance

DR. WESLEY IAN

DISCLAIMER

The information in this book is not meant to replace professional medical advice, diagnosis, or treatment; rather, it is meant mainly for general informational reasons. If you have any questions about a medical problem, you should always consult your doctor or another trained health expert. Don't ever discount expert medical advice or put off getting it because of something you've read in this book.

Any negative effects or repercussions arising from the usage of the material provided herein are not the responsibility of the book's author or publisher. It should be noted by readers that the material in this book is not all-inclusive and might not address every facet of the subject. Furthermore, new research may have an impact on how health concerns are understood or treated because medical knowledge is always changing.

No particular test, treatment, method, or product mentioned in this book is endorsed or promoted by the author or publisher. The reader assumes all risk associated with using the information included in this book.

Before making any big decisions regarding your health, it's crucial to speak with a licensed healthcare provider. The relationship between a patient and their healthcare practitioner should not be replaced by this book, nor is it meant to offer medical advice.

The opinions presented in this book are the author's and may not necessarily represent those of the publisher. Any errors, omissions, or inaccuracies in the information in this book are not the responsibility of the author or publisher.

It is recommended that readers independently confirm any information contained in this book and speak with a healthcare provider about their specific medical needs and state of health.

TABLE OF CONTENTS

ABOUT THE BOOK

"Navigating Tongue Tie with Confidence and Care" is an invaluable tool for parents, caregivers, and medical professionals who want an in-depth understanding of the intricate world of tongue knots. An informative introduction sets the stage for an examination of the many facets of this illness in the book's first section. The author, who most likely has a degree in medicine, provides a comprehensive explanation of tongue tie that includes its definition, anatomy, types, causes, and risk factors. The comprehension of the condition's nuances by readers is contingent upon their grasp of this fundamental understanding.

The vital field of diagnosis and evaluation is explored. Common misdiagnoses are discussed, along with how to recognize tongue ties in infants, the significance of getting professional assistance, and diagnostic instruments and processes. The book delves into the emotional and psychological effects of tongue tie, going beyond its clinical elements. The author guides the reader through the issues of parental worry, anxiety, and the impact on nursing, speech development, and the child's emotional health.

The book explores the available treatment alternatives, including post-procedure care, alternative therapies, and an explanation of the idea of frenotomy (tongue-tie release). The book does a great job of leading readers through the decision-making process by highlighting the need to make educated decisions, working with healthcare specialists, comprehending possible outcomes, and taking long-term ramifications into account.

The focus of the book shifts to useful support strategies. "Supporting Breastfeeding" offers priceless advice on overcoming obstacles, finding lactation resources and assistance, and perfecting positioning methods for both pumping and bottle-feeding. "Speech and Language Development" examines milestone tracking, speech therapy's role, exercises, activities, and long-term development considerations all at the same time.

In its concluding section, it presents a comprehensive approach to tongue tie that incorporates integrative methods including bodywork and therapy, dietary modifications, stress and anxiety reduction, and the establishment of a nurturing atmosphere. With its abundance of knowledge, the book presents itself as an invaluable resource, giving readers the skills and assurance necessary to handle the complications of tongue tie with caution and assurance.

CHAPTER ONE

INTRODUCTION TO TONGUE TIE

RECOGNIZING TONGUE TIE

The lingual frenulum, a band of tissue located beneath the tongue, is abnormally short or tight, causing tongue tie, also known as ankyloglossia, a condition that impairs tongue movement. This illness can show in numerous ways, impacting an individual's ability to execute specific oral activities, such as speaking, eating, and even breastfeeding. To fully comprehend tongue tie, one must investigate its definition, the anatomy involved, the various varieties that can occur, as well as its causes, risk factors, and the critical responsibility of identifying its symptoms.

DEFINITION AND ANATOMY

A tongue knot is characterized by the restricted movement of the tongue produced by a shortened or tight lingual frenulum. The lingual frenulum is a band of tissue that connects the underside of the tongue to the floor of the mouth. In individuals with tongue ties, this band is abnormally short or tight, limiting the range of motion of the tongue. This restriction can impact various oral functions, such as articulating sounds, eating, and breastfeeding.

Understanding the normal anatomy of the lingual frenulum and its role in tongue movement is essential in comprehending the challenges faced by those with this condition.

TYPES OF TONGUE TIE

Tongue tie is not a one-size-fits-all condition, as different types vary in severity. Classifying tongue tie is often based on the extent to which the lingual frenulum restricts the movement of the tongue. The classification includes anterior tongue tie, where the frenulum is attached close to the tip of the tongue, and posterior tongue tie, where the attachment is farther back on the tongue. The severity of the restriction can also be classified into mild, moderate, or severe, depending on the extent to which it limits the tongue's movement.

REASONS AND DANGER ELEMENTS

The exact causes of tongue tie are not always clear, but several factors may contribute to its development. One primary factor is believed to be genetic, with tongue ties often running in families. Additionally, certain environmental factors during fetal development may contribute to the condition. Research suggests that a combination of genetic and environmental factors may increase the likelihood of a child being born with a tongue tie. Other risk factors include conditions such as Ehlers-Danlos syndrome and certain medications taken during pregnancy.

RECOGNIZING SYMPTOMS

Identifying the symptoms of tongue tie is crucial for early intervention and management. In infants, common signs include difficulty latching during breastfeeding, leading to feeding challenges for both the baby and mother. As a child grows, speech difficulties may become apparent, with issues such as difficulty pronouncing certain sounds or a persistent speech impediment. Beyond infancy and childhood, untreated tongue ties can lead to various challenges in adulthood, such as difficulty with oral hygiene practices and potential social and psychological impacts related to speech impediments.

A comprehensive understanding of tongue tie involves delving into its definition, the intricate anatomy associated with the condition, the various types that exist, as well as the causes, risk factors, and the importance of recognizing symptoms for timely intervention. By gaining insight into these facets of tongue-tie, individuals, caregivers, and healthcare professionals can work collaboratively to address the challenges posed by this condition and enhance the quality of life for those affected.

CHAPTER TWO

DIAGNOSIS AND ASSESSMENT

IDENTIFYING TONGUE TIES IN INFANTS

Identifying tongue ties in infants is a crucial aspect of early childhood development and can significantly impact various facets of a child's health. Tongue tie, or ankyloglossia, occurs when the strip of skin beneath the baby's tongue (lingual frenulum) is shorter than usual, limiting the range of motion. This condition can affect a baby's ability to breastfeed effectively, impacting both their nutrition and the bonding experience with their mother. Identification of tongue tie often involves observing signs such as difficulty latching onto the breast, shallow sucking, and maternal nipple pain during breastfeeding.

SEEKING PROFESSIONAL HELP

Seeking professional help is imperative when concerns arise regarding tongue ties in infants. Consulting with healthcare professionals, such as pediatricians, lactation consultants, or ear, nose, and throat (ENT) specialists, can provide a comprehensive assessment. These experts can evaluate the baby's feeding patterns, observe physical symptoms, and consider the mother's experiences to determine whether intervention is necessary. Seeking timely professional help ensures that any potential issues associated with tongue tie are addressed promptly, promoting the overall well-being of both the infant and the mother.

DIAGNOSTIC TOOLS AND PROCEDURES

Diagnostic tools and procedures play a pivotal role in the accurate assessment of tongue ties in infants. Healthcare professionals employ a variety of methods to diagnose the condition, including visual inspection, physical examination, and assessment of feeding dynamics. In some cases, specialized tools, such as a tongue depressor or a screening tool like the Hazelbaker Assessment Tool for Lingual Frenulum Function may be utilized to evaluate the degree of restriction. Diagnostic procedures may also involve considering the overall health of the infant, as tongue tie can sometimes be associated with other medical conditions.

COMMON MISDIAGNOSES

Despite the importance of accurate diagnosis, there are instances of common misdiagnoses related to tongue tie in infants. Misinterpretation of normal variations in anatomy or overlooking subtle signs can lead to either underdiagnosis or overdiagnosis of tongue ties. Professionals may mistakenly attribute feeding difficulties to tongue tie without considering other factors, or conversely, they may overlook the condition in cases where it is present.

Additionally, the subjective nature of some symptoms, such as maternal pain during breastfeeding, can contribute to misdiagnoses. Healthcare providers need to approach the assessment of tongue tie with a comprehensive and nuanced understanding, considering the unique circumstances of each infant and their mother to avoid unnecessary interventions or overlooking genuine concerns.

CHAPTER THREE

EMOTIONAL AND PSYCHOLOGICAL IMPACT

PARENTAL CONCERNS AND ANXIETY

Parental concerns and anxiety play a pivotal role in shaping the emotional and psychological well-being of both parents and children. The transition to parenthood often brings about a range of worries related to the child's health, safety, and overall development. These concerns can be intensified by societal expectations, personal experiences, and the plethora of information available through various sources. Anxiety, when left unaddressed, may hinder the parent-child relationship and impact the child's emotional development.

Creating a supportive environment that fosters open communication and seeks professional guidance can help alleviate parental concerns and contribute to a healthier emotional climate for both parents and children.

IMPACT ON BREASTFEEDING

Breastfeeding is a fundamental aspect of early childhood development with profound emotional and psychological implications. The ability to breastfeed fosters a unique bond between the mother and child, providing not only essential nutrients but also emotional comfort and security. However, challenges such as difficulties with latch, inadequate milk supply, or maternal stress can significantly impact the breastfeeding experience. These challenges may contribute to feelings of inadequacy and frustration for the mother, potentially affecting her emotional well-being. Supportive interventions, including lactation counseling and emotional support, are crucial in addressing breastfeeding-related concerns and fostering a positive emotional connection between the mother and child.

EFFECTS ON SPEECH DEVELOPMENT

Speech development is a critical milestone in a child's cognitive and emotional growth. Parental interactions and the overall emotional environment play a key role in shaping a child's language acquisition and communication skills. When parents experience heightened anxiety or face challenges in providing a nurturing communication environment, it can potentially impact the child's speech development. Children may mirror the emotional states of their caregivers, and a tense atmosphere can hinder their confidence in expressing themselves verbally.

Creating a positive and supportive atmosphere, engaging in interactive communication, and seeking early intervention if needed are essential strategies to promote healthy speech development and emotional well-being in children.

EMOTIONAL WELL-BEING OF THE CHILD

The emotional well-being of a child is intricately linked to various factors, including parental influences, early experiences, and overall family dynamics. Parental concerns and anxieties, if not effectively managed, can create an emotional ripple effect on the child. Children often absorb and reflect the emotional climate around them, making it crucial for parents to prioritize their mental health and seek support when needed. A secure and nurturing environment, characterized by love, understanding, and effective communication, lays the foundation for a child's emotional well-being. Recognizing and addressing any signs of emotional distress in the child, such as changes in behavior or mood, is essential for fostering a positive and resilient emotional foundation that will serve them well into adulthood.

CHAPTER FOUR

OPTIONS FOR TREATMENT

FRENOTOMY (TONGUE TIE RELEASE)

Frenotomy, commonly known as tongue tie release, is a medical procedure performed to address a condition called ankyloglossia, where the strip of skin beneath the tongue (lingual frenulum) is shorter than usual, restricting the range of motion. This condition, often present at birth, can interfere with various oral functions, such as breastfeeding, speech, and oral hygiene. Frenotomy involves cutting the frenulum to release the tongue's movement, allowing for improved functionality. The procedure is typically a quick and relatively simple intervention that can be performed in various healthcare settings.

ALTERNATIVE THERAPIES

Alternative therapies are approaches that some individuals explore either as complements to traditional medical treatments or as primary interventions. In the context of ankyloglossia, alternative therapies may include exercises and stretches aimed at improving tongue mobility, chiropractic adjustments, or myofunctional therapy.

However, individuals must consult with healthcare professionals to ensure that chosen alternative therapies are safe and effective. While some may find relief or improvement through alternative methods, the evidence supporting their efficacy in treating tongue tie is often limited, and their use should be approached with caution.

POST-PROCEDURE CARE

Post-procedure care following a frenotomy is essential for optimal recovery. Parents and caregivers of infants who undergo the procedure are typically advised to engage in gentle stretching exercises to prevent the reattachment of the frenulum. Proper oral hygiene practices, such as keeping the area clean, may also be recommended. In some cases, pain management strategies for the infant, such as the use of over-the-counter pain relievers, may be suggested. Follow-up appointments with the healthcare provider are crucial to monitor the healing process and address any concerns that may arise.

RISKS AND BENEFITS

As with any medical procedure, there are both risks and benefits associated with frenotomy. The primary benefit is the potential improvement in oral functions, particularly in cases where ankyloglossia is causing difficulties with breastfeeding, speech development, or oral hygiene. However, like any surgery, there are inherent risks, including bleeding, infection, and the possibility of the frenulum reattaching, requiring additional intervention.

It is essential for healthcare providers to thoroughly discuss these risks and benefits with patients or parents, ensuring they have a clear understanding of what to expect before making informed decisions about the procedure.

Frenotomy is a medical intervention that addresses the challenges posed by tongue tie, with the potential to significantly improve oral functions. While alternative therapies may be considered, they should be approached with caution and in consultation with healthcare professionals. Post-procedure care is crucial for a successful recovery, and understanding the associated risks and benefits is essential for making informed decisions about the intervention.

CHAPTER FIVE

NAVIGATING THE DECISION-MAKING PROCESS

INFORMED DECISION-MAKING

Informed decision-making is a critical aspect of navigating the complex landscape of choices that individuals encounter in various facets of life. Whether it pertains to personal matters, professional endeavors, or healthcare decisions, being informed empowers individuals to make choices that align with their values and preferences. In the context of healthcare, informed decision-making involves acquiring relevant information about potential treatments, their associated risks and benefits, and understanding the implications of various options.

WORKING WITH HEALTHCARE PROFESSIONALS

Working with healthcare professionals is integral to the informed decision-making process, as these professionals possess the expertise needed to guide individuals through complex medical information. Collaborative discussions with healthcare providers foster a better understanding of diagnoses, available treatment options, and the potential impact of those choices on one's health. Establishing effective communication with healthcare professionals ensures that individuals can ask questions, seek clarification, and actively participate in the decision-making process, thereby contributing to a more patient-centered approach to care.

UNDERSTANDING POTENTIAL OUTCOMES

Understanding potential outcomes is a crucial component of the decision-making journey. It involves a realistic assessment of the various scenarios that may unfold based on the choices made. In healthcare, this entails grasping the potential benefits and drawbacks of different treatment options, considering the likelihood of success, and being aware of any potential complications. This understanding enables individuals to weigh the risks and benefits, aligning their decisions with their personal values, goals, and the level of risk they are willing to accept.

CONSIDERING LONG-TERM IMPLICATIONS

Considering long-term implications adds a strategic dimension to decision-making, encouraging individuals to think beyond immediate outcomes. Whether it's a healthcare decision or any other life choice, contemplating the long-term consequences involves forecasting how decisions may impact one's life, health, and overall well-being over an extended period. In healthcare, this may involve assessing the potential for treatment side effects, the need for ongoing medical interventions, and the impact on quality of life in the long run.

Navigating the decision-making process involves a holistic approach that incorporates informed decision-making, collaboration with healthcare professionals, understanding potential outcomes, and considering long-term implications. By embracing these concepts, individuals can make decisions that are not only well-informed but also aligned with their values and conducive to their overall well-being. The integration of these principles facilitates a more thoughtful and intentional decision-making process across various aspects of life, contributing to a more fulfilling and purposeful journey.

CHAPTER SIX

ENCOURAGEMENT OF BREASTFEEDING

OVERCOMING OBSTACLES IN BREASTFEEDING

Encouraging breastfeeding is essential for moms' and babies' health and well-being. For many mothers, overcoming breastfeeding obstacles is a typical issue, and fostering effective breastfeeding experiences requires proper assistance. The first pain or discomfort that some women may feel when nursing is one major obstacle. Correct positioning of the baby at the breast and instruction on good latch methods can help with this.

RESOURCES AND ASSISTANCE FOR LACTATION

Furthermore, lactation assistance and resources are essential in helping moms through the process of nursing. Healthcare experts with expertise in lactation assistance, known as lactation consultants, can offer individualized advice to address particular issues and difficulties.

The network of resources accessible to nursing moms is further enhanced by access to community-based support groups, internet forums, and instructional materials. This creates a welcoming environment where women may share their experiences and seek advice from others.

TECHNIQUES FOR POSITIONING

It is essential to use positioning strategies when breastfeeding to guarantee efficient milk transfer and avoid frequent problems like nipple discomfort and insufficient milk production. Mothers need to know how to latch their babies correctly, how to place them, and how important it is to provide a calm and comfortable nursing environment. It is possible to experiment with different techniques like the football hold, cradle hold, and side-lying posture to determine which one works best for mother and child.

STRATEGIES FOR PUMPING AND BOTTLE-FEEDING

Pumping and bottle-feeding techniques become crucial for moms who might have to be taken from their babies or who struggle with direct breastfeeding. With the help of breast pumps, moms can express their milk, preserving their supply and enabling others to assist with feeding. To support milk production, it is critical to educate mothers on the safe and effective use of breast pumps, how to store expressed milk, and the need to stick to a regular pumping schedule.

Strategies for bottle-feeding also contribute to the support of nursing moms. It's important to take the baby's age, nursing status, and personal preferences into account before introducing a bottle. To minimize the possibility of nipple confusion and facilitate a seamless transition from the breast to the bottle, slow-flowing nipples, and timed bottle-feeding techniques can assist in replicating the natural nursing experience.

Promoting breastfeeding entails several approaches, such as overcoming obstacles, offering lactation support and resources, highlighting appropriate positioning methods, and teaching moms efficient pumping and bottle-feeding procedures. Communities can help breastfeeding programs succeed by identifying the special needs of each mother-infant pair and creating a supportive atmosphere that benefits the health and well-being of both moms and newborns.

CHAPTER SEVEN

DEVELOPMENT OF SPEECH AND LANGUAGE

KEEPING AN EYE ON MILESTONES

It is essential to track speech and language development milestones to comprehend and assist a child's communication skills. These benchmarks offer a structure for evaluating a child's development and pointing out possible red flags. Parents and other caregivers are essential in noticing and recording these developmental milestones, from the early cooing and babbling stages to the emergence of first words and sentences. Frequent monitoring makes it possible to identify speech and language impairments early on and provide assistance and intervention promptly.

SPEECH-LANGUAGE PATHOLOGY

For people who are having trouble communicating, speech therapy is a useful tool. A range of strategies are used by speech-language pathologists, sometimes known as speech therapists, to treat particular issues with articulation, fluency, voice, and language abilities. These experts collaborate closely with people of all ages, customizing their interventions to suit each person's needs. Speech therapy attempts to increase a person's capacity for effective self-expression and to improve general communication skills through focused exercises and activities.

ACTIVITIES AND EXERCISES

In both everyday life and therapeutic contexts, exercises and activities are essential to the development of speech and language. Play-based activities help children learn and express language more effectively. By exposing kids to a diverse linguistic environment, simple activities like reading books, constructing blocks, or imaginative play promote language development.

Speech therapy exercises are controlled, repetitive tasks that reinforce desired communication abilities to treat specific issues, such as articulation or language comprehension.

EXTENDED-TERM ASPECTS

Recognizing that communication is a dynamic and ever-evolving process is important for long-term thinking in speech and language development. Individuals' communication requirements and capacities can vary as they move through different phases of life.

It is critical to take into account how speech and language development affects social relationships, academic performance, and general well-being. Long-term planning may include solutions for resolving communication difficulties in a variety of life contexts, modifications in educational settings, and continued speech therapy support.

Key components of promoting healthy speech and language development include milestone monitoring, speech therapy participation, engaging in pertinent exercises and activities, and taking long-term ramifications into account. Caregivers, educators, and speech therapists all play a vital role in improving people's communication skills and general well-being by remaining aware of their unique requirements and offering appropriate solutions.

TONGUE TIE: HOLISTIC METHODS THAT COMBINE BODYWORK AND THERAPY

When it comes to treating tongue ties, holistic methods offer a diverse viewpoint that extends beyond conventional medical procedures. An essential component of this comprehensive approach is the integration of bodywork and therapy. Understanding the relationship between the mind, body, and emotions, practitioners can alleviate constraints and tensions underlying tongue knots by using bodywork treatments like craniosacral therapy or myofascial release.

By encouraging an increased range of motion, restoring equilibrium within the musculoskeletal system, and assisting the body's natural healing processes, these therapy methods seek to improve overall well-being.

NUTRITIONAL ASPECTS

An important component of holistic therapy for tongue ties is dietary concerns. The body's growth and development depend heavily on nutrition, and dietary decisions can affect dental health. Holistic doctors might look into dietary changes that promote the best possible development and function of the tongue. In a holistic approach, a focus on nutrient-dense foods that support general health and tissue healing can be essential. Moreover, dietary therapies might be designed to target specific inadequacies that may aggravate tongue tie or make it more difficult to resolve.

CONTROLLING ANXIETY AND STRESS

An additional crucial element of a comprehensive strategy for treating tongue tie is managing stress and anxiety. Physical health is greatly influenced by emotional well-being, and tightness in the muscles that control tongue function can be a symptom of stress and anxiety. Holistic methods to address emotional variables that may cause or worsen tongue ties include mindfulness exercises, relaxation methods, and therapy. Holistic approaches try to establish an atmosphere that is supportive of general health and well-being by encouraging emotional balance and resilience.

ESTABLISHING A HELPFUL ENVIRONMENT

The cornerstone of treating tongue ties holistically is establishing a supportive atmosphere. This entails encouraging an all-encompassing and cooperative strategy that takes into account the person as well as their local environment. To treat people with tongue ties holistically, family dynamics, cultural considerations, and social support networks are essential. Holistic professionals can collaborate with families to establish a setting that promotes candid dialogue, comprehension, and assistance during the recovery phase. To guarantee a comprehensive and patient-centered approach, this may entail counseling, education, and cooperation with other medical specialists.

Holistic methods for treating tongue ties acknowledge the complex interactions of environmental, psychological, and physical elements. Managing stress and anxiety, taking into account nutritional factors, combining massage and therapy, and fostering a supportive atmosphere all contribute to a comprehensive framework that goes beyond discrete medical treatments. These holistic methods aim to maximize general well-being by treating the person as a whole and provide a more integrative and holistic approach to tongue-tie treatment.